PREFACE

My name is Valencia Annik Payne, BSN, RN, BS, Biology. I received my BS in Nursing from Delta State University and my BS in Biology from Jackson State University. I am a former Navy PACU RN that has instructed and tutored many nursing students, as well as, many Registered Nurses. As an Author of Fluid and Electrolytes for Nursing Students, I feel that nursing students should have the condensed "what you need to know" nursing content. This book is designed to simplify what you need to know about fluid and electrolytes and will help the students perform well on their classroom tests, HESI, and NCLEX. I hope you all enjoy this visual aid or guide on Fluid and Electrolytes.

CONTENTS

FLUID AND ELECTROLYTES

POTASSIUM

MAGNESIUM

PHOSPHORUS

CALCIUM

SODIUM

Normal Electrolyte Ranges

Na (Sodium): 135-145 mEq/L

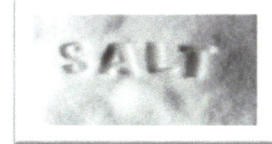

K (Potassium): 3.5-5.0 mEq/L

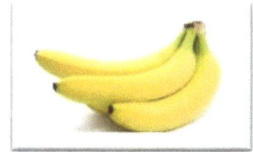

Ca (Calcium): 9.0-10.5 Mg/dl

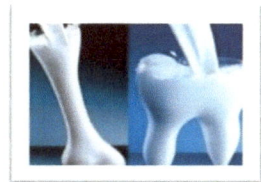

Mg (Magnesium): 1.2-2.1 mEq/L

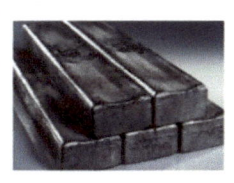

HYPERVOLEMIA: FLUID VOLUME EXCESS (FVE)

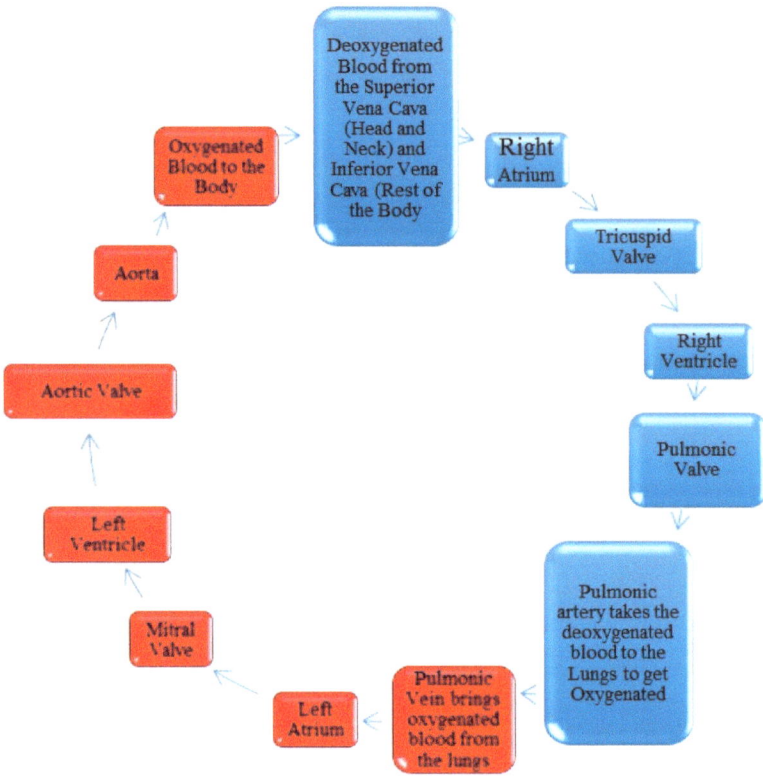

PROBLEM WITH THE HEART!!!!!

TIP: ALWAYS REMEMBER THE BLOOD FLOW OF THE HEART

TIP: The Mitral Valve is also known as the Bicuspid!!!!

REMEMBER THIS PHRASE: You Have to Try (Tricuspid Valve) Before You Buy (Bicuspid or Mitral Valve)

SIGNS AND SYMPTOMS OF FVE

1. Increase Volume means Increase Pressure

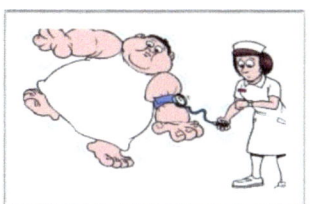

2. Increase pulse

3. Distended neck veins and peripheral veins

4. Peripheral edema called 3rd spacing: vessels cannot retain that much fluid so they begin to leak

5. Lung sounds are wet

6. Any acute weight loss or gain is due to fluid

Question: How does the body try to remove this excess fluid?

Answers: 1. Polyuria: kidneys are helping you to diuresis or remove the excess fluid

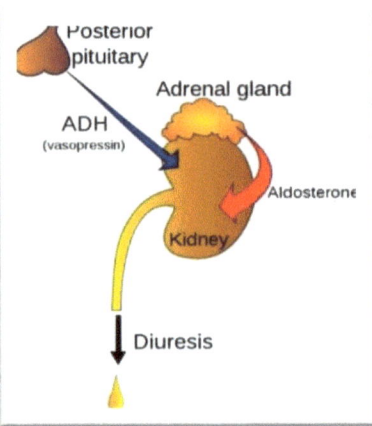

2. Weeping of skin: Due to excess fluid overload, the skin is stretched tightly and it becomes thin and the interstitial fluid seeps or weeps out through the pores.

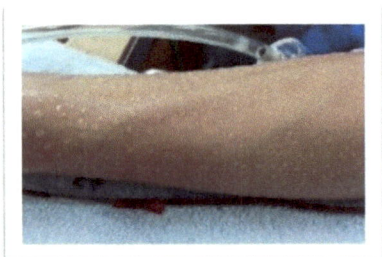

CAUSES CONGESTIVE HEART FAILURE

Right Sided Heart Failure

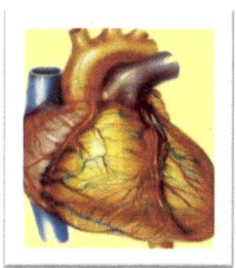

A. Decreased Cardiac Output

B. Decreased Urine Output

C. Decreased Kidney Perfusion that causes Renal Failure

Left Sided Heart Failure

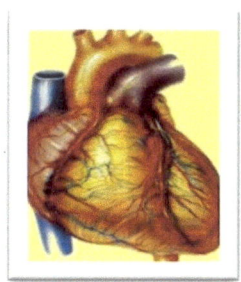

A. Fluid buildup in the lungs

B. Shortness of Breath (SOB)

TREATMENTS

1. Lasix: Loop diuretic
2. HCTZ (Hydrochlorothiazide)
3. Aldactone (Potassium Sparing Diuretic)

INTERVENTION

1. Diuresis is induced by bed rest
   A. Why: Lying supine you perfuse your kidneys more because of increase cardiac output.

FLUID VOLUME DEFICIT

CAUSES

1. Loss of fluid from any area of the body

Example: vomiting, hemorrhage, and Paracentesis

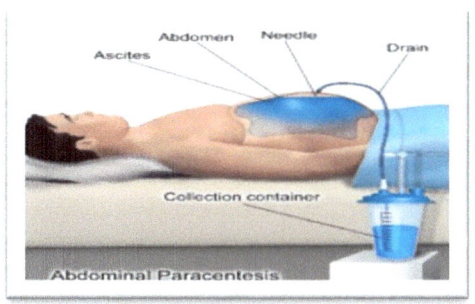

2. **3rd Spacing**: Fluid is in a place that is not effective for the patient
    Examples: Ascites and burns

3. Diseases that include polyuria

4. Nasogastric tube hooked to suction

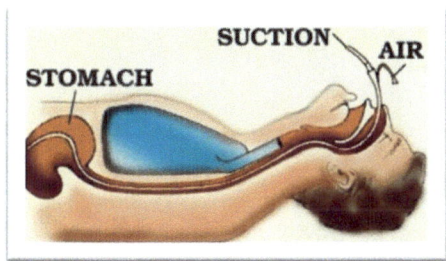

SIGNS AND SYMPTOMS

1. Dry mucous membranes

2. Decrease urine output
   Why: Kidneys are not being perfused

3. Decrease skin turgor

4. Decrease blood pressure: Low Volume equals Low Pressure

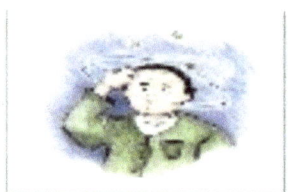

5. Increase heart rate
   Why: Because the heart is trying to pump what little is left in circulation

6. Decrease central venous pressure: Low Volume equals Low Pressure

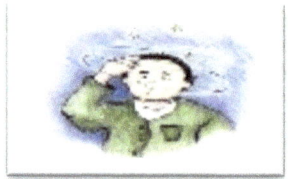

7. Flat peripheral veins/neck veins

8. Cool extremities
   Why: Because the blood is being shunted to vital organs

9. Urine specific gravity is increased: If the patient is putting out any urine it will be concentrated

TREATMENTS AND INTERVENTIONS

Mild FVD: Give PO (BY MOUTH) fluids

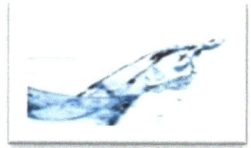

Severe FVD: Give IV fluids

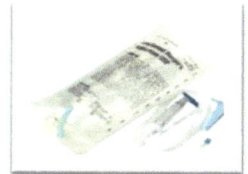

INTRAVENOUS FLUID

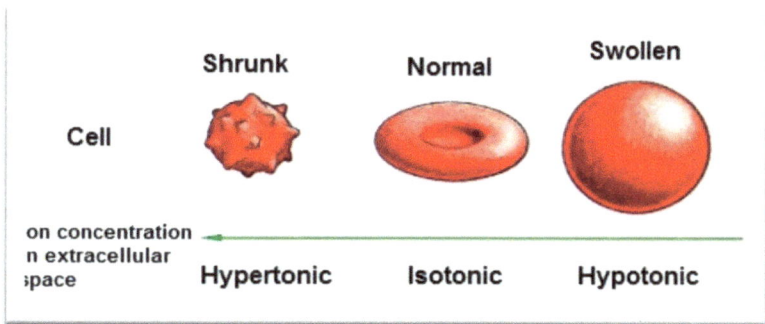

Isotonic Solution: Goes into the vascular space and remains there

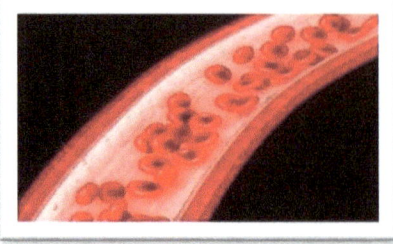

<u>Example</u>: Normal Saline (NS), Lactate Ringers (LR), and D5W

Hypertonic Solution: Solution that draws water out of the cell and places it in the vascular space

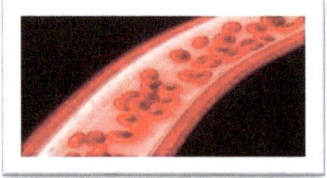

<u>Example</u>: D10W, 5%NaCl, D5 ½ NaCl, TPN, D5NaCl, D5LR, and 3%NaCl

Hypotonic Solution: Solution causes fluid to leave the vascular space and enter the cells. The cell will swell and lyse

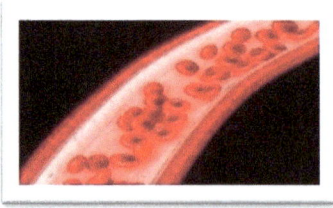

<u>Example</u>: D2.5W, ½ NaCl, and 0.33% NaCl

HYPERMAGNESIUM: SEDATIVE EFFECT

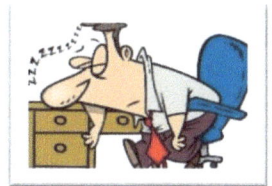

KIDNEYS EXCRETE MAGNESIUM

CAUSES

1. Renal Failure

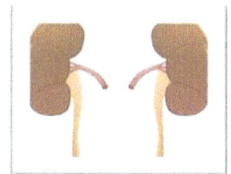

2. Antacids

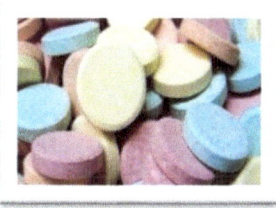

3. Flushing

4. Warmth

5. Magnesium will make you vasodilate

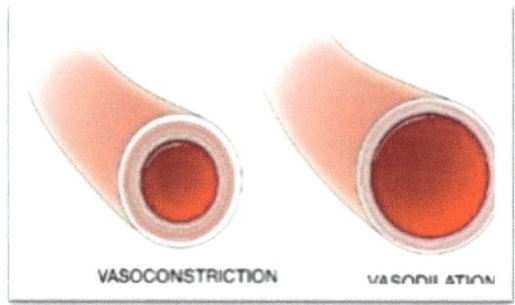

SIGNS AND SYMPTOMS

1. Decreased or absent Deep Tendon Reflexes

2. Arrhythmias and Asytsole

3. Decreased Level of Consciousness (LOC)

4. Decreased Pulse

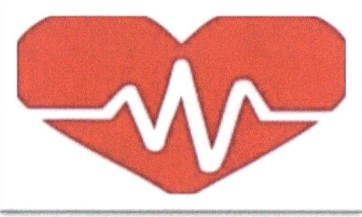

5. Decreased Respirations

6. Muscle Tone (Decreased)

TREATMENT

1. Administer Calcium Gluconate ***IV PUSH SLOWLY***:
    In the presence of Mg, they cancel each other out.

2. Dialysis

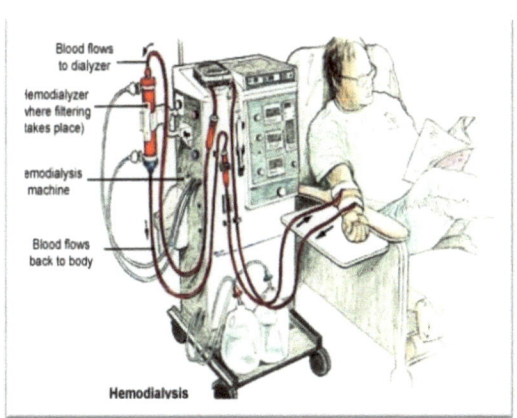

3. Ventilator

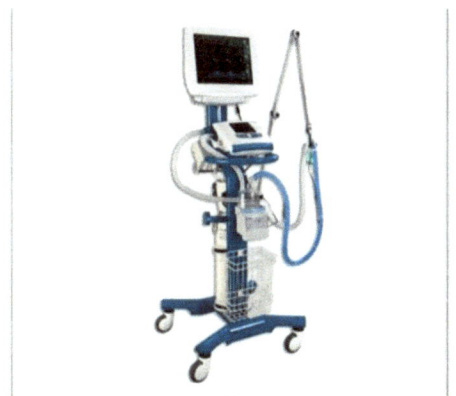

HYPERCALCEMIA: SEDATIVE EFFECT

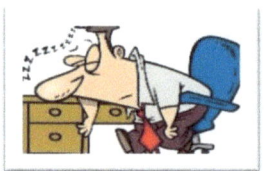

1. Kidney stones are mostly made up of Calcium

2. Taking thiazides (Retain Calcium)

3. Hyperparathyroidism : Too much PTH

4. Immobilization

5. Soft bones

SIGNS AND SYMPTOMS

1. Decreased or absent Deep Tendon Reflexes

2. Muscle Tone (Decreased)

3. Arrhythmias or Asystole

4. Decreased Level of Consciousness (LOC)

5. Decreased Pulse

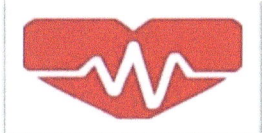

6. Decreased Respirations

TREATMENTS

1. Get up and move

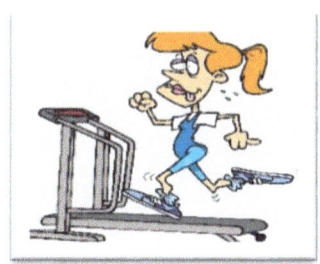

2. Give them fluids

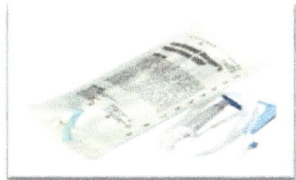

3. Calcium has an inverse relationship with Phosphorous

   A. When Phosphorous is UP Calcium is DOWN

   B. When Phosphorous is DOWN Calcium is UP

4. Steroids cause Calcium to GO DOWN

    A. Long term use of steroids causes osteoporosis

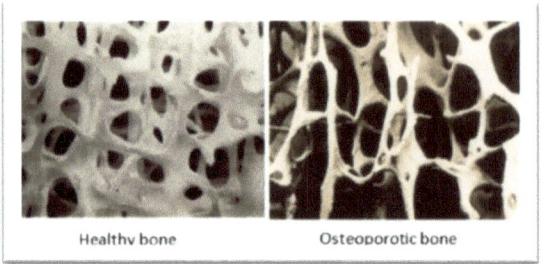

Healthy bone   Osteoporotic bone

5. Diet: Anything with Protein and Phosphorus

6. Need Vitamin D

7. Vitamin D lives on the skin and is activated by the:

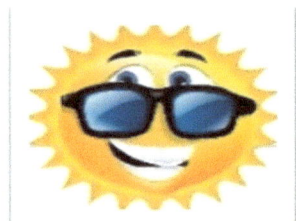

8. Calcitonin decreases Serum Calcium

HYPOMAGNESIUM: NO SEDATIVE

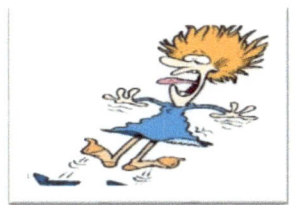

CAUSES

1. Diarrhea: Magnesium lost in the intestines

2. Alcohol is hypertonic and makes you diuresis

    A. Suppresses ADH (Anti-Diuretic Hormone)

3. Not eating foods that containing Magnesium

SIGNS AND SYMPTOMS

1. Muscle tone (Rigid and Tight)

2. Seizure

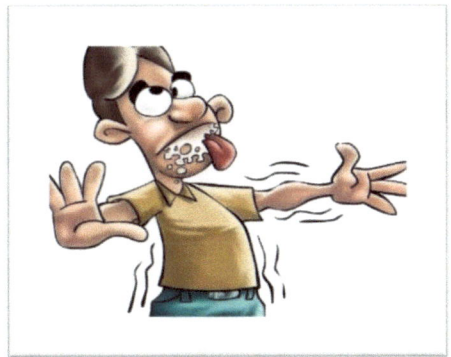

3. Muscle Spasms or Cramps

4. Muscle Weakness (Airway, Heart, and Esophagus are muscles)

5. Increased Deep Tendon Reflexes

6. Change in mental status

7. + Chvostek's = Tap Cheek

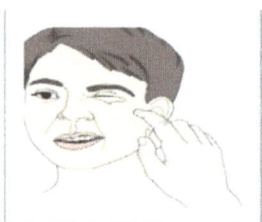

8. Positive (+)Trousseau's = Pump up BP cuff

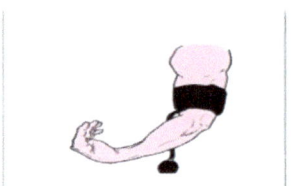

TREATMENTS

1. Give Magnesium Levels

2. Check kidney function before and during IV magnesium

Question

During an IV Mg infusion, your patient starts sweating and flushing. As a nurse what will you do?

Answer

STOP THE INFUSION!!!!!!!

HYPOCALCEMIA: NO SEDATIVE

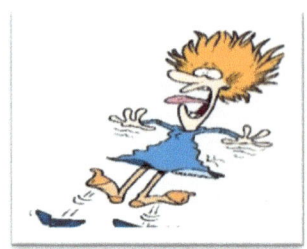

CAUSES

1. **Thyroidectomy**: The removal of all or part of your thyroid gland. Your thyroid is a butterfly-shaped gland located at the base of your neck. It produces hormones that regulate your metabolism.

2. **Hypoparathyroidism**: An uncommon condition in which your body secretes abnormally low levels of parathyroid hormone (PTH). PTH plays an important role in regulating and maintaining a balance of your body's levels of two minerals: calcium and phosphorus.

3. **Radical Neck Dissection**: Metastatic neck disease is the most important factor in the spread of head and neck squamous cell carcinoma from primary sites. The primary sites most commonly involved in the spread of this carcinoma are the mucosal areas of the upper digestive tract. These include the larynx, oropharynx, hypopharynx, and oral cavity.

SIGNS AND SYMPTOMS

1. Muscle tone (Rigid and Tight)

2. Seizures

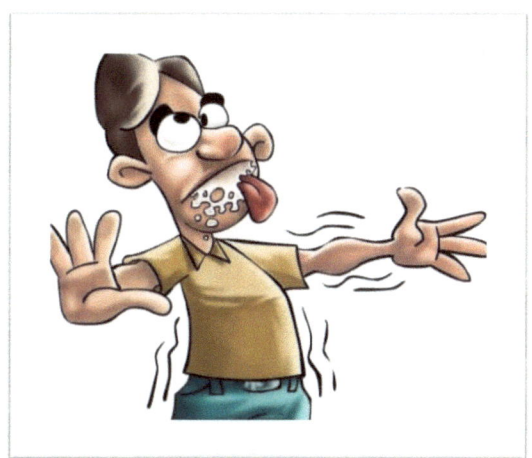

3. Muscle Spasms or Cramps

4. Muscle Weakness (Airway, Heart, and Esophagus are

   muscles)

5. Increased Deep Tendon Reflexes

6. Change in mental status

7. Positive (+) Chvostek's = Tap Cheek

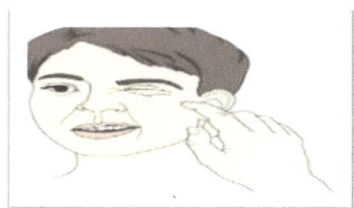

8.   + Trousseau's = Pump up BP cuff

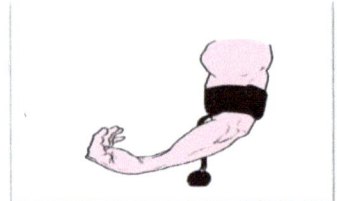

TREATMENTS

1. Give Vitamin D

2. IV Ca2+: Make sure the patient is on a heart monitor while getting IV Ca2+
    If you see a widen QRS on the monitor STOP THE INFUSION!!!!!!

3. **Phosphorous binding agents**: Aluminum salts, Calcium Carbonate, and Calcium Acetate

HYPERNATREMIA: TOO MUCH SODIUM AND NOT ENOUGH H$_2$O

SODIUM CHANGES=NEUROLOGICAL CHANGES

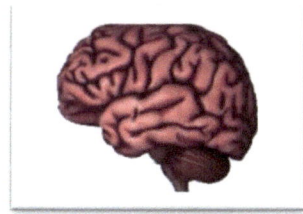

WATER FOLLOWS SODIUM

CAUSES

1. **Hyperventilation**: Due to insensible water loss (evaporative water loss from the respiratory tract).

2. Heat stroke

3. **Diabetes Insipidus**: is a condition that is caused by excessive thirst (polydipsia) and excretion of large amounts of diluted urine (polyuria).

SIGNS AND SYMPTOMS

1. Dry mouth

2. Thirsty

3. Swollen Tongue (Late Sign)

TREATMENTS

1. Restrict Na+

2. Dilute patient with IV fluids

3. DECREASED serum Na+ = Dilution

4. Daily weights

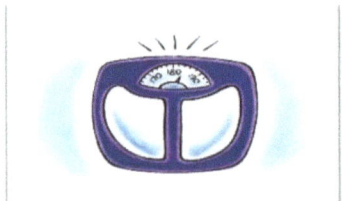

5. Intake and Output

6. **Patients with feeding tubes will get dehydrated**: Because the patients have fluid and electrolyte imbalances that are associated with their underlying disease process.

HYPONATREMIA: TOO MUCH H_2O AND NOT ENOUGH SODIUM

SODIUM CHANGES=NEUROLOGICAL CHANGES

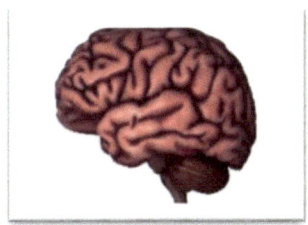

CAUSES

1. Vomiting or sweating: Drinking H_2O only replaces H_2O and dilutes the blood.

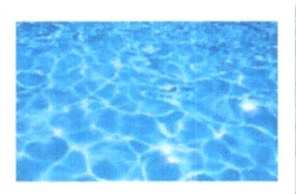

2. D5W (Sugar and Water)

3. SIADH (Syndrome of Inappropriate ADH secretion): TOO MUCH ADH

   A Lot of Letters = A Lot of Water

   1. Urine decreased and concentrated

   2. Blood is diluted

   3. Dealing with Na+ specific gravity lab: Dilution make the numbers GO DOWN and Concentration make the numbers GO UP

Psychogenic Polydipsia: In love with drinking H_2O and this causes Na+ shift in the brain and gives them a high

TREATMENTS

1. Patient is in need of Na+

2. Do not give patient H_2O

3. If neuro problems are on board then give patient a hypertonic solution

HYPERKALEMIA

LIFE THREATENING ARRHYTHMIAS

K+ IS EXCRETED BY THE KIDNEYS; WHEN THE KIDNEYS ARE NOT
FUNCTIONING PROPERLY THE SERUM K+ GOES UP

CAUSES

1. Kidney Issues

2. Aldactone: Drug makes the patient retain potassium

SIGNS AND SYMPTOMS

Muscle twitching+ weakness+ flaccid paralysis

TREATMENTS

1. Dialysis: Due 2 nonfunctioning of the kidneys

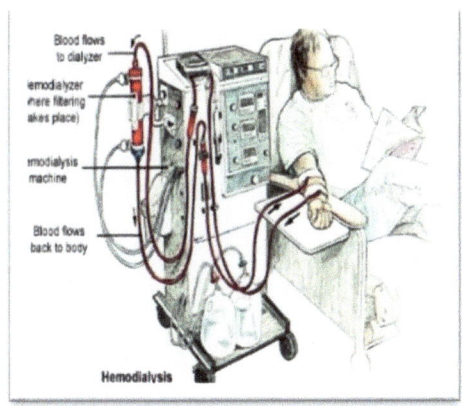

2. Calcium gluconate decreases arrhythmias

3. Glucose ($C_6H_{12}O_6$) and Insulin

   A. Insulin brings along glucose and potassium into the cell

   B. When you give IV insulin, your concern will be hypokalemia and hypoglycemia

4. Kayexalate: Given to treat Hyperkalemia

   A. Exchanges Na+ for K+ in the GI tract. The patient excretes the K+ (potassium) thru BOWEL MOVEMENT.

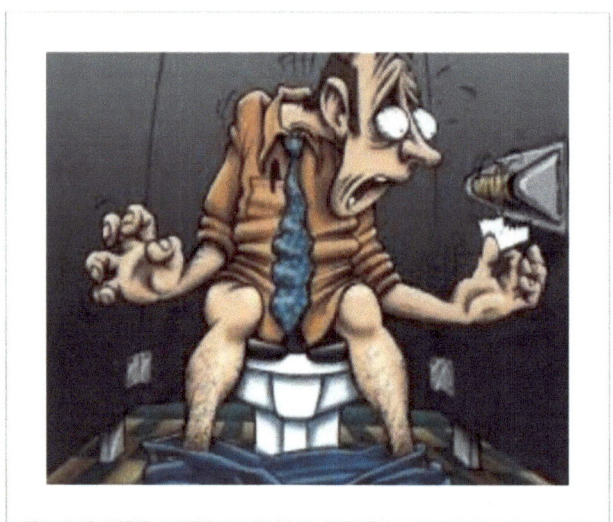

HYPOKALEMIA

LIFE THREATENING ARRHYTHMIAS

CAUSES

1. Vomiting

2. NG Suction

3. Diuretics

4. Not eating the proper foods that contain K+

SIGNS AND SYMPTOMS

1. Muscle Cramps

2. Muscle Weakness

TREATMENTS

1. Give potassium IV or PO

2. **Aldactone**: Drug that makes you retain potassium

3. Eat potassium: Bananas, Oranges, Bake Potatoes, and Avocados

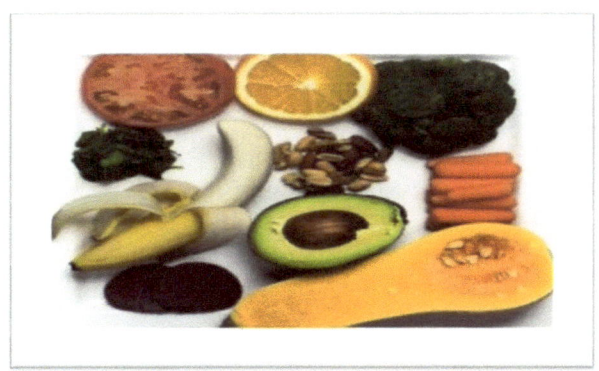

ALDOSTERONE (STEROID MINERALCORTICOID)

1. Aldosterone is in the adrenal glands

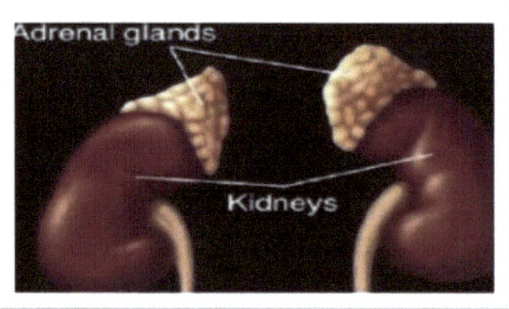

2. Mechanism of Action

   A. If the blood volume gets low due to hemorrhage or vomiting, aldosterone is secreted to retain $Na+$ and H_2O to increase blood volume

3. Diseases that contain too much aldosterone

   A. **Cushing Disease**: Caused by a tumor on the pituitary gland. The pituitary gland releases too much ACTH (Adrenocorticotropic hormone). ACTH stimulates production and release of cortisol which is a stress hormone. Too much ACTH causes the adrenal glands to make too much cortisol.

   B. **Hyperaldosteronism**: Too much aldosterone is produced by the adrenal glands. This can cause lower levels of potassium in the blood (hypokalemia).

4. Disease that contain too little aldosterone

   A. **Addison Disease**: The adrenal glands are not making enough cortisol or aldosterone.

ADH (ANTI-DIURETIC HORMONE): RESIDES IN THE PITUITARY

1. If you see these key words in your test questions: Any Head Injuries, Craniotomy, and Sinus Surgeries *THINK PROBLEM WITH ADH*

2. Vasopressin is an ADH drug

NCLEX PRACTICE QUESTIONS

1. The client is admitted to the unit with a potassium level of 2.2 mEq/L. The client with this potassium level will display which symptoms?

   A. Muscle rigidity
   B. Peaked T waves
   C. Rapid respirations
   D. U waves

2. The client is admitted to the hospital with hypokalemia. An IV of normal saline 40ml with 20 mEq of potassium chloride is infusing. Prior to the beginning the infusion, the nurse will:

   A. Check the calcium level
   B. Check the magnesium level
   C. Check the creatinine level
   D. Check the sodium level

3. The client in the labor and delivery unit has preeclampsia. IV magnesium is infusing on the pump. Which of these findings will indicate hypermagnesium?

   A. Absence of the knee-jerk reflex
   B. Blood pressure of 150/80
   C. Respirations of 30 per minute
   D. Urinary output of 60 ml/hr

4. The client that has Cushing disease will exhibit signs of:

   A. Hypermagnesium
   B. Hypocalcemia
   C. Hypernatremia
   D. Hypokalemia

NCLEX PRACTICE QUESTIONS

5. The nurse is responsible for teaching the client the proper dietary choices to obtain magnesium. Which food is a good source of magnesium?

   A. Liver
   B. Apple
   C. Squash
   D. Spinach

6. The client that has hyperparathyroidism will have which electrolyte imbalance?

   A. Hyponatremia
   B. Hyperphosphatemia
   C. Hypokalemia
   D. Hypercalcemia

7. An elderly client is admitted to the unit with a temperature of 102.2. The client has a urinary specific gravity of 1.032 and dry tongue. The should anticipate a doctor's order for:

   A. A diuretic
   B. An antibiotic
   C. An IV of normal saline
   D. An analgesic

NCLEX ANSWERS

1. **D is the correct**
   Rationale: Answer A is incorrect because the muscles will be flaccid. Answer B is incorrect because that is an indication of an elevated potassium level. Answer C is incorrect because the respirations will be shallow.

2. **C is the correct**
   Rationale: The client receiving IV potassium will need renal function evaluated prior to infusion. Answers A, B, and D are incorrect because these levels do not need to be checked prior to infusion.

3. **A is correct**
   Rationale: The signs of magnesium toxicity are respirations less than 12 breathes per minute, oliguria, and absence of deep tendon reflexes. Answer B is incorrect because the blood pressure is within normal limits. Answer C is incorrect because the respirations will have to be below 12 breathes per minute. Answer D is incorrect because the urinary output is within normal limits.

4. **C is correct**
   Rationale: The client has a hyperadrenal function which causes the retention of sodium and water. Answers A, B, and D are incorrect because the client don't usually lose magnesium, potassium, or calcium.

5. **D is correct**
   Rationale: Green leafy vegetables and legumes contain a high amount of magnesium. Answers A, B, and C are incorrect because they do not provide exceptionally significant sources of magnesium.

6. **D is correct**
   Rationale: The client will have elevated calcium levels because the calcium is pulled from the bone into the serum. Answers A, B, and C are incorrect because the client will not have hyponatremia, hypocalcemia, or hyperphosphatemia.

7. **C is correct**
   Rationale: The client is suffering from hypovolemia and hyponatremia. The elevated temperature is related to dehydration and the urinary specific gravity shows urinary concentration. Answers A, B, and D are incorrect because further data in the question is not available.

REFERENCES

Berkowitz, A. (2007). *Clinical pathophysiology made ridiculously simple*. Miami, FL: MedMaster Inc.

Ignatavicius, D., & Workman, M. (2006). *Medical-Surgical Nursing critical thinking for collaborative care*. Saint Louis, Missouri: Elsevier Saunders.

PHOTO CREDITS

http://blog.timesunion.com/opinion/blaming-the-parents-is-premature-wrong/8837/human-brain-on-white-background-2/

http://www.thevirtualnephrologist.com/mobile/dialysis-g8.html

http://www.healthable.org/how-to-keep-track-of-your-heart-rate/

http://toonclips.com/design/6787

http://galleryhip.com/oh-no-cartoon.html

http://www.psycheducation.org/mechanism/8StressHormones.htm

http://quizlet.com/18971944/chapter-10-notes-by-paula-flash-cards/

http://medical-dictionary.thefreedictionary.com/Trousseau's+sign

http://stock-free-images.com/image/wallpaper-of-underwater-coral

http://www.allthingsdiscussed.com/More/Isotonic-hypertonic-and-hypotonic-solutions.php

http://en.wikipedia.org/wiki/Paracentesis

http://www.qmedicine.co.in/top%20health%20topics/E/epilepsy%20general.html

http://www.phun.no/?p=225

http://www.ashleysweeneyrd.com/belly-bloat/

https://thedetoxteacompany.com.au/free-sample/

http://www.instah.com/diabetes/what-is-polyuria/

http://fittedkitchendesign.com/cartoon-bunk-bed/

http://www.waiting.com/nasogastric.html

http://www.blickman.com/products/541110100

www.ingramcontent.com/pod-product-compliance
Lightning Source LLC
Chambersburg PA
CBHW050842180526
45159CB00004B/1992